FERTILITY BREAKTHROUGH:

Harnessing the Power of Egg Quality for Pregnancy

DR. ANNETTE E. SPENCER

DISCLAIMER

TABLE OF CONTENT

Table of Contents

DISCLAIMER 2

INTRODUCTION 6

UNLOCKING THE SECRETS OF
FERTILITY 6

1. Opening Quote or Prologue 7

Prologue: A Symphony of Hope 8

1. Author's Note 8

CHAPTER 1 11

THE SCIENCE BEHIND EGG QUALITY 11

3.1 EGG DEVELOPMENT AND MATURATION 13

*The Ballet of Creation: Unveiling the Stages of Egg
Development* 13

The Crucial Maturation Phase: 19

3.2 GENETIC AND EPIGENETIC INFLUENCES
....21

Decoding the Genetic Symphony: The Role of Genetics in
Egg Quality: 22

Genetic Determinants of Egg Quality: 23

Impact of Age on Egg Quality: 24

FERTILITY BREAKTHROUGH

Epigenetic Factors: The Dance of Environmental Influence...........25

CHAPTER 2...........28

NUTRITION AND LIFESTYLE FOR OPTIMAL EGG QUALITY...........28

2.1 THE ROLE OF NUTRITION...........29

Embarking on the Fertility Feast:...........30

Fertility-Boosting Tips:...........35

4.2 LIFESTYLE MODIFICATIONS...........38

The Fertility Symphony:...........38

READER-CENTRIC SOLUTIONS: NAVIGATING CHALLENGES WITH EASE.42

CHAPTER 3...........46

HOLISTIC APPROACHES TO ENHANCE EGG QUALITY...........46

3.1 MIND-BODY CONNECTION...........47

READER'S REFLECTION: MAKING THE MIND-BODY CONNECTION TANGIBLE...........51

3.2 ALTERNATIVE THERAPIES...........54

Reader's Exploration: A Personalized Holistic Journey.....58

CHAPTER 4...........62

ADVANCED FERTILITY TECHNOLOGIES AND TREATMENTS...........62

4.1 ASSISTED REPRODUCTIVE TECHNOLOGIES (ART) 64

Reader's Perspective: Understanding and Embracing ART 67

6.2 EGG FREEZING AND PRESERVATION 69

READER'S CONSIDERATION: NAVIGATING CHOICES FOR FUTURE FERTILITY...72

CHAPTER 5 76

SUCCESS STORIES AND REAL-LIFE EXPERIENCE 76

5.1 PERSONAL TESTIMONIALS 77

Reflection: Finding Hope in Shared Experiences 81

5.2 EXPERT INSIGHTS..83

Reader's Inquiry: Navigating Questions and Seeking Answers 86

CONCLUSION 89

SUMMARIZE KEY TAKEAWAYS......................90

INTRODUCTION

UNLOCKING THE SECRETS OF FERTILITY

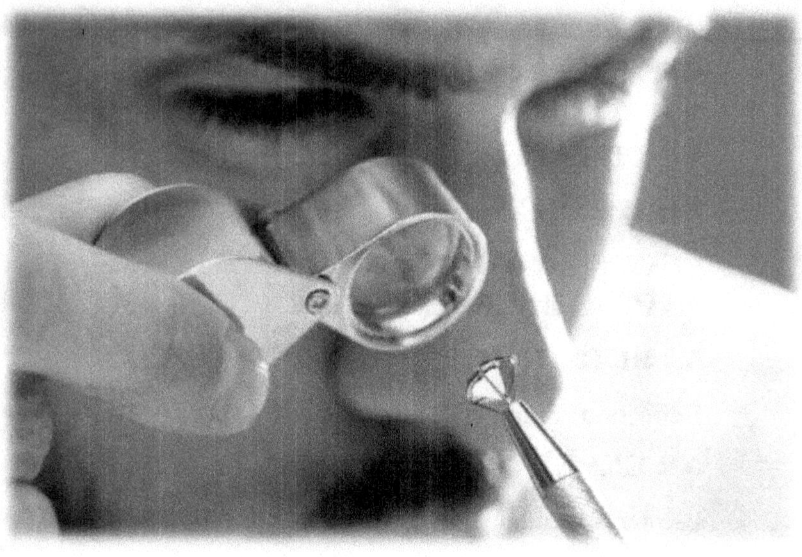

In the path of making life, the nuances of fertility frequently stay cloaked, shrouded in mystery. This chapter serves as the entryway to

unlocking those mysteries, bringing forth the significant relevance of egg quality in the reproductive narrative.

1. Opening Quote or Prologue

"In the delicate dance of fertility, hope is the music that leads us."

These words resound through the hallways of this inquiry into fertility, setting the tone for a trip that intertwines science, emotion, and the resilience of the human spirit. Alternatively, let me share a touching prologue that draws you into the life of a couple dealing with the complications of fertility.

Prologue: A Symphony of Hope

In a tiny room where the aroma of sterilized surroundings lingers, Mark and Sarah find themselves engaged in a dance that is both beautiful and heartbreaking. As they negotiate the rollercoaster of reproductive treatments, the echoes of hope and anguish ricochet within the walls. Their tale is merely one note in the symphony of many couples yearning for the melody of a new life. In their fight, we find the heartbeat of many.

In their resilience, we find the universal human experience of desire, resilience, and the hunt for solutions. As we begin on this journey together, let Mark and Sarah's narrative be a compass, leading us across the terrain of fertility breakthroughs.

1. Author's Note

Dear Reader, Welcome to a tale that goes beyond medical vocabulary and clinical processes. As the author of this inquiry into fertility breakthroughs, I provide not only data but a genuine relationship to the subject matter. It is a relationship created from personal experiences, from observing the hardships and achievements of those close to me, and from a passionate dedication to shine light on the transforming potential of understanding and enhancing egg quality. In the mosaic of life, fertility serves as a cornerstone.

My motivation for authoring these lines originates from the realization that the quality of this foundation dramatically impacts the tapestry of one's life. Perhaps you, like me, have felt the weight of uncertainty on this path.

It is my deepest intention that inside these pages, you discover not only information but a guiding light, a source of hope, and a reservoir of knowledge that helps you to negotiate the challenges of fertility.

This book is more than a collection of chapters; it is a roadmap constructed with empathy, scientific precision, and a touch of the human spirit. As you peruse the pages, may you discover the transformational breakthroughs you seek, and may the mysteries of fertility be disclosed, one revelation at a time.

With compassion and understanding,
[Dr. Annette E. Spencer]

CHAPTER 1

THE SCIENCE BEHIND EGG QUALITY

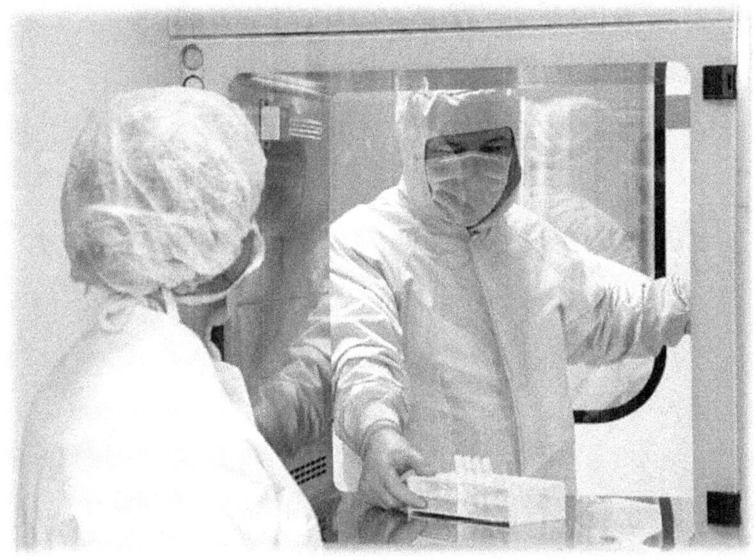

In the delicate dance of conception,

knowing the scientific basis of egg

quality becomes crucial. This

chapter looks into the complex tapestry of egg development, uncovering the genetic and epigenetic forces that define the delicate journey toward conception.

3.1 EGG DEVELOPMENT AND MATURATION

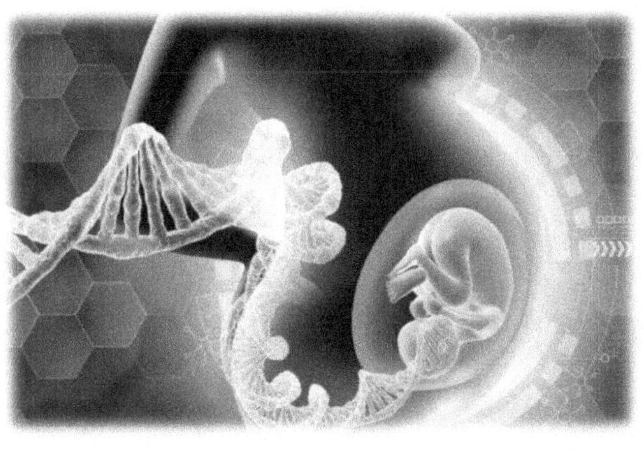

The Ballet of Creation: Unveiling the Stages of Egg Development :The path toward conception starts with the intriguing process of egg formation.

Picture this as a ballet, where each movement is choreographed with precision and purpose. In the early stages, primordial follicles emerge from dormancy, signifying the commencement of a transforming dance.

Primary Growth Phase: Nurturing the Seedlings As the primordial follicles commence on the route of growth, they enter the main growth phase. This period is comparable to the fostering of seedlings in the soil foundational and vital. The granulosa cells encircling the developing egg coordinate its growth, setting the scene for the complicated performance ahead.

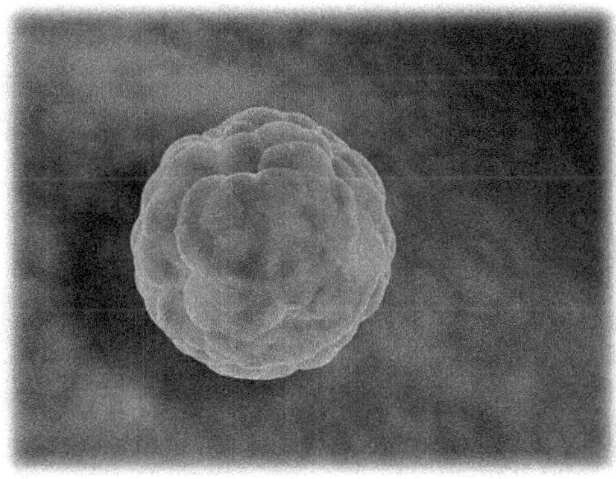

Secondary Growth: The Unfurling of Potential Secondary development represents a critical moment in this ballet, where the eggs undergo major alterations. The follicles continue to expand, and a fluid-filled cavity forms, enclosing the mature egg. This phase reflects the unfurling of petals, unveiling the promise within. Antral

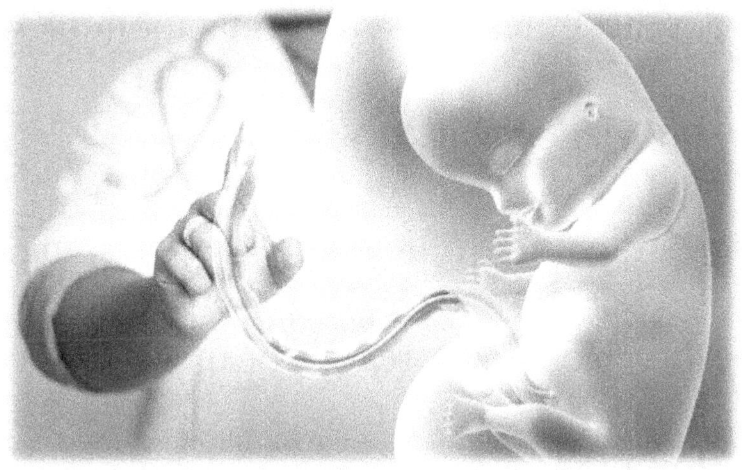

Follicle Stage: The Ensemble Takes Shape Like an ensemble of dancers rehearsing for a spectacular performance, the antral follicles grow. Each follicle harbors one egg, and the interaction between hormones orchestrates the synchronization of this delicate ensemble. The dominating follicle appears, marking the lead dancer ready for the limelight.

Ovulation: The Grand Finale

Ovulation, the grand finale of this dance, is the result of rigorous preparation. The main dancer the mature egg is liberated from its follicular cocoon, ready to take center stage. This moment, coordinated with the menstrual cycle, contains the secret to fertility.

The Crucial Maturation Phase:

Determining Egg Quality Within this ballet of growth, the maturation period emerges as the cornerstone. The quality of the egg during ovulation greatly determines the fertility story. Explore the elements that lead to proper maturation and the relevance of this period in the hunt for conception.

Understanding the complexity of egg formation lays the stage for appreciating the science underlying egg quality. Visual aids and analogies can be applied to increase clarity, ensuring that readers appreciate the balletic grace of this biological

journey.

3.2 GENETIC AND EPIGENETIC

INFLUENCES

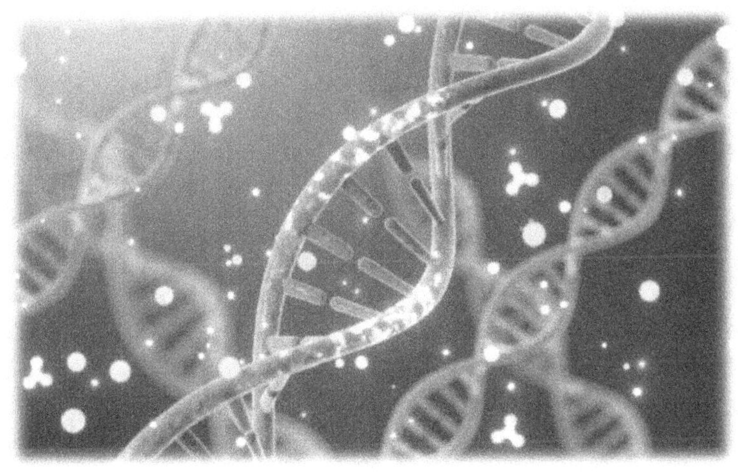

Decoding the Genetic Symphony: The Role of Genetics in Egg Quality: Genetics, the silent director of the biological symphony, plays a vital role in molding egg quality. Unravel the complicated strands of genetic impact, reducing sophisticated topics for reader understanding.

Genetic Determinants of Egg Quality:

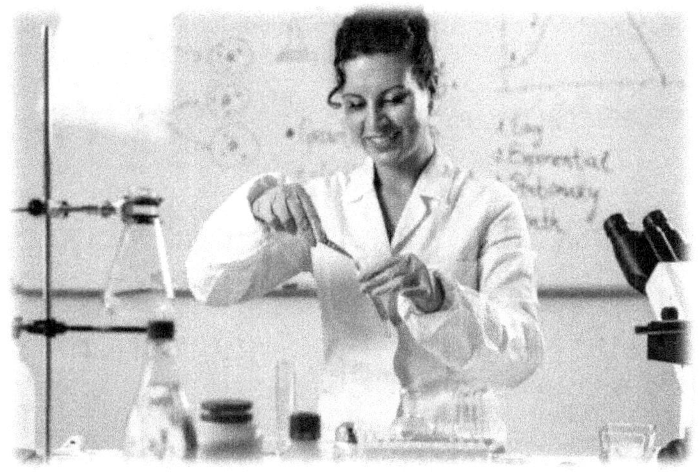

Delve into the genetic elements that contribute to egg quality. Explore the function of chromosomal integrity, stressing the significance of a balanced chromosomal makeup for optimal fertility.

Impact of Age on Egg Quality:

Address a critical element impacting genetics the age of the egg carrier. Explain how age affects the genetic material within eggs, offering light on the obstacles and possibilities connected with fertility at different life stages.

Epigenetic Factors: The Dance of Environmental Influence

As the genetic score plays out, the dance of epigenetic variables takes center stage. These extrinsic impacts on gene expression add a degree of intricacy to the reproductive tale.

Defining Epigenetics for the Lay Reader: Break down the notion of epigenetics, explaining how external stimuli impact gene activity without modifying the underlying DNA sequence. Analogies can be applied to simplify this sophisticated biological process.

Environmental factors and epigenetic dance: Explore the contextual forces that affect the epigenetic dance. From lifestyle decisions to exposure to pollutants, describe how external variables might affect the genetic expression of eggs.

By demystifying the genetic and epigenetic impacts on egg quality, this chapter gives readers the core information needed to navigate the complexity of fertility. Visual aids, analogies, and real-life examples increase the accessibility of this scientific investigation.

CHAPTER 2

NUTRITION AND LIFESTYLE FOR OPTIMAL EGG QUALITY

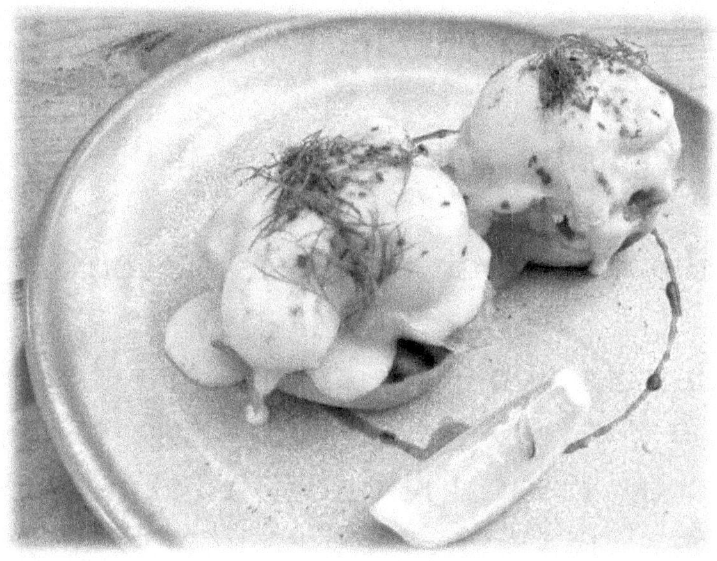

In the complicated dance of fertility,

diet and lifestyle emerge as

choreographers, sculpting the delicate

performance of egg health. This chapter unravels the relevance of what we consume and how we live in the hunt for maximum egg quality.

2.1 THE ROLE OF NUTRITION

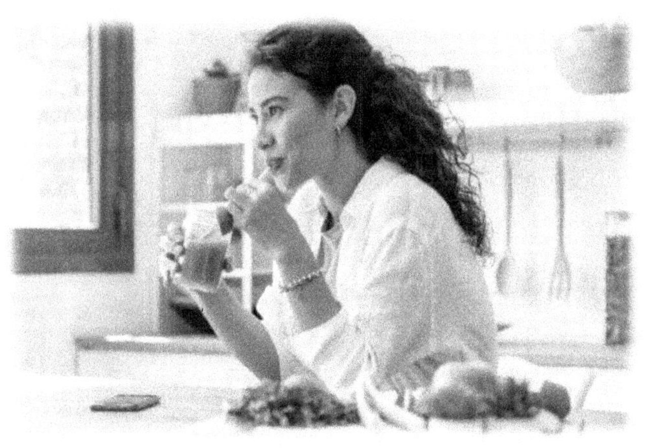

Embarking on the Fertility Feast: The Impact of Nutrition on Egg Health Picture nutrition as the symphony playing in the background of the fertility ballet a harmonic composition that impacts the whole performance. Delve into the tremendous influence of nutrition on egg quality, breaking down complicated topics into manageable parts.

Essential Nutrients for Egg Health:

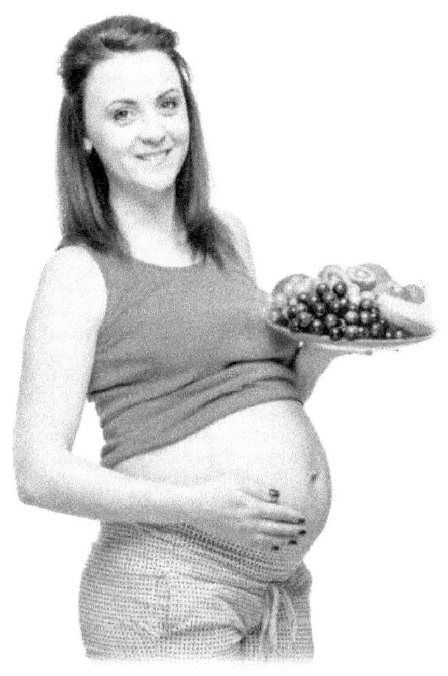

Navigate the world of fertility-friendly foods. From antioxidants to omega-3 fatty acids, examine the building blocks that contribute to good egg health. Provide a thorough list of fertility-boosting foods, each having a distinct function in nourishing the delicate dance of conception.

Navigating the Micronutrient Maze:

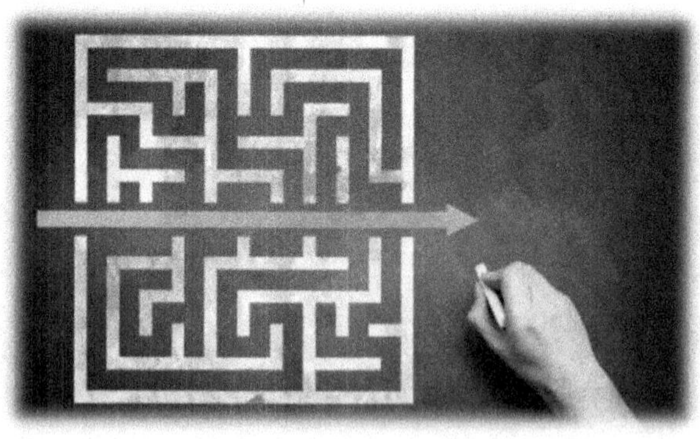

Micronutrients, the unsung heroes of the fertility tale, need a spotlight. Illuminate the significance of vitamins and minerals in supporting egg quality. Employ analogies and related examples to boost reader understanding.

The Culinary Canvas: Crafting a Fertility-Boosting Meal Plan

Translate nutritional knowledge into practical recommendations. Offer a sample meal plan meant to encourage fertility, making it easier for readers to adopt these ideas into their daily lives. Infuse creativity into the culinary canvas, making the road toward optimum egg health a tasty experience.

Fertility-Boosting Tips: A Pocket Guide for Readers

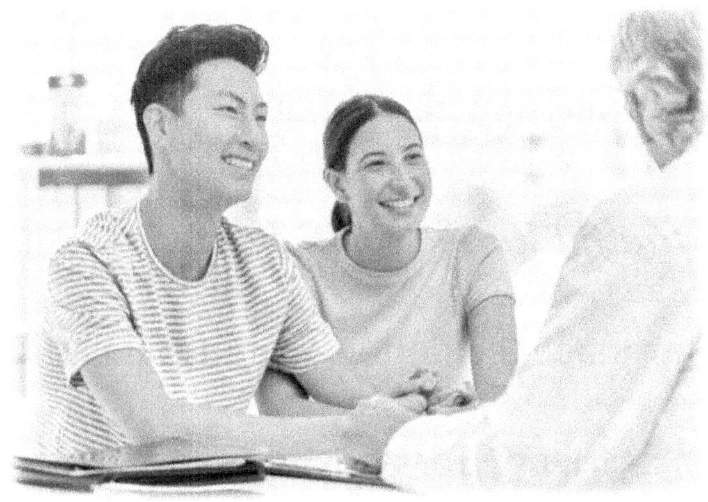

Hydration Habits: The Elixir of Fertility Explore the often-overlooked function of water in fertility. Illustrate how proper water intake leads to

good egg health, drawing

comparisons between hydration and

the nourishment of fragile blossoms.

Mindful Eating for Fertility:

Introduce the notion of mindful eating

as a strategy for boosting fertility.

Discuss the significance of enjoying

each food, establishing a stronger

connection with the nutritional

journey.

The Power of Balance: Moderation and Variety Highlight the significance of a balanced diet. Discuss the significance of moderation and diversity in ensuring that the fertility feast is both nutritious and pleasant.

By infusing this section with practical recommendations, realistic examples, and a touch of culinary inventiveness, readers will go on a sensory journey

of nutrition's influence on fertility.

4.2 LIFESTYLE

MODIFICATIONS

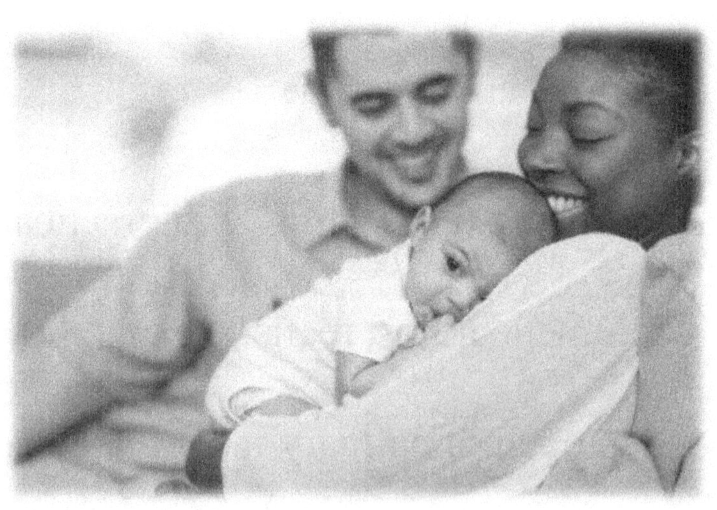

The Fertility Symphony: Harmonizing Lifestyle and Conception Beyond the sphere of diet, lifestyle takes the stage, impacting the crescendo of fertility. This section addresses practical lifestyle improvements that positively impact the reproductive narrative.

Stress Management: Orchestrating Serenity in the Fertility Ballet Stress, the quiet disruptor of the fertility ballet, demands careful control. Dive into actionable stress-reduction approaches, from mindfulness practices to relaxation exercises. Offer real-life anecdotes, making the message relevant and motivating.

Soothing Slumber: The Dance of Sleep and Fertility Unveil the relationship between sleep and conception, showing appropriate rest as the soft lullaby leading the fertility journey. Provide recommendations for enhancing sleep quality and managing common sleep issues.

Movement as Medicine: The Dance of Physical Activity Celebrate the significance of physical exercise in maintaining optimum fertility. From the rhythmic dance of yoga to the exhilarating steps of strolling, learn exercise techniques that enhance reproductive health.

READER-CENTRIC SOLUTIONS: NAVIGATING CHALLENGES WITH EASE

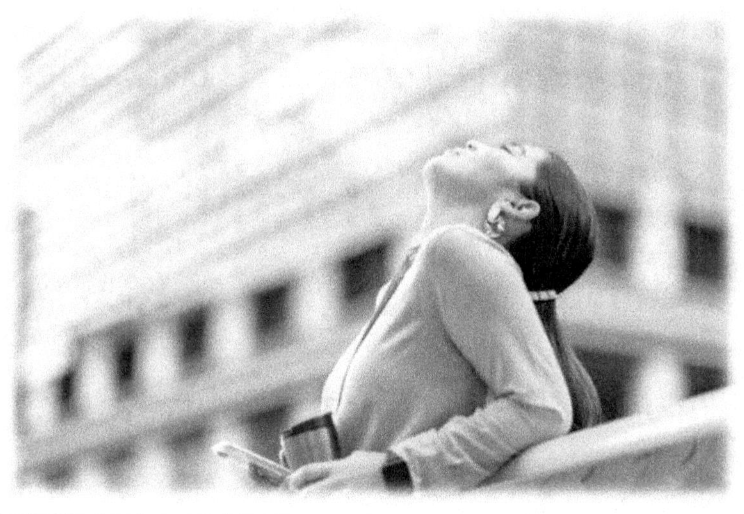

Realistic Approaches to Stress Management: Acknowledge the reality of contemporary living and give reasonable techniques for stress

management. Encourage readers to

incorporate doable tactics into their

routines.

The Art of Prioritizing Sleep:

Recognize the obstacles to sleep in a

hectic society. Provide

recommendations for prioritizing

sleep, stressing quality over quantity,

and addressing frequent sleep

disruptors.

Incorporating Joyful Movement:

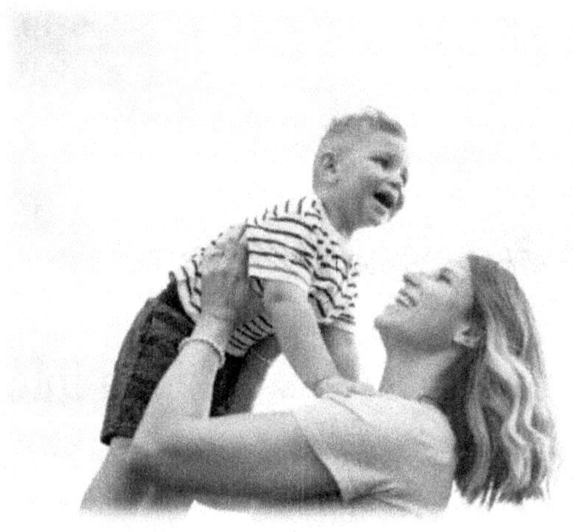

Emphasize the joy of movement.

Showcase varied physical activities,

inviting readers to select the dance

that connects with their particular inclinations.

By addressing lifestyle alterations in a reader-centric manner, this section attempts to empower individuals on their reproductive journey. It offers a combination of science-backed ideas and practical solutions, establishing a path for improving both diet and lifestyle for maximum egg quality.

CHAPTER 3

HOLISTIC APPROACHES TO ENHANCE EGG QUALITY

In the complicated tapestry of fertility, holistic methods emerge as threads weaving across the mind, body, and spirit. This chapter begins on a voyage into the realms of the holistic, studying how the mind-body connection and alternative therapies might be used to boost egg quality.

3.1 MIND-BODY

CONNECTION

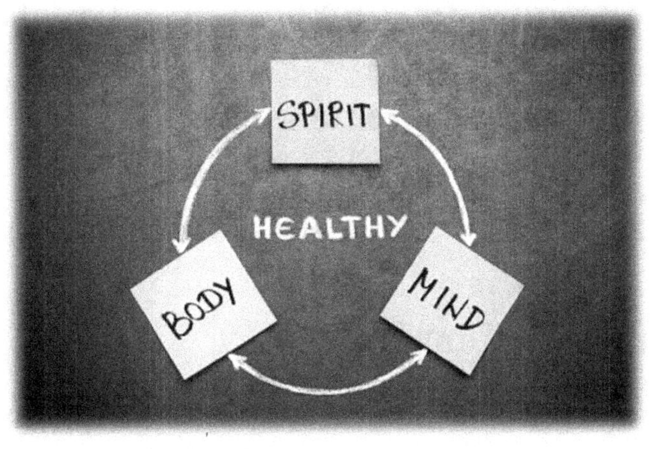

Harmony Within: Nurturing Mind-Body Synchrony

Understanding the Mind-Body Link:

Embark on an examination of the

complicated link between mental well-being and fertility. Use understandable language to illustrate the ways in which emotions, stress, and mentality may impact the delicate dance of conception.

Mindfulness: A Symphony of Presence Introduce mindfulness as a key technique for boosting egg quality. Explore the practice of being present in the moment and its favorable influence on reproductive health. Share relevant tales or case studies that show the transforming power of mindfulness.

Relaxation Techniques:

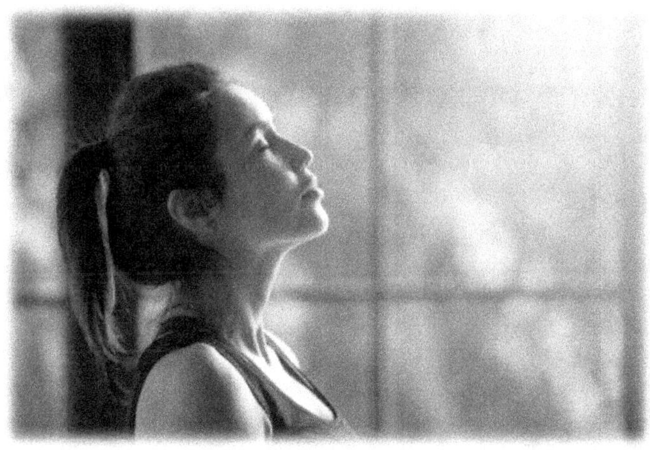

The Gentle Waltz to Conception Dive into numerous relaxation techniques, from deep breathing to gradual muscular relaxation. Illustrate how these strategies may be smoothly integrated into daily life, acting as a relaxing backdrop to the reproductive quest.

READER'S REFLECTION: MAKING THE MIND-BODY CONNECTION TANGIBLE

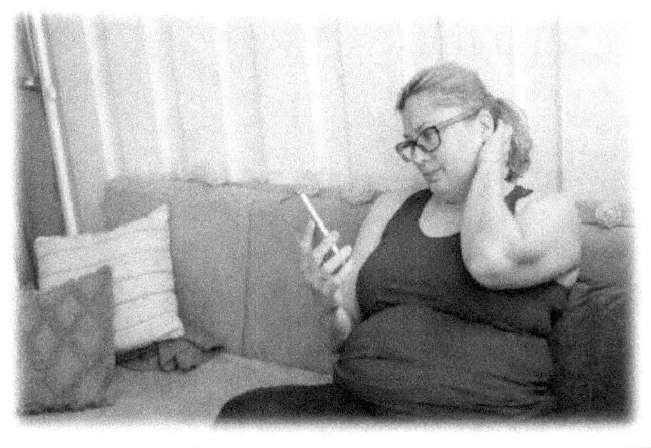

Practical Mindfulness in Everyday

Life: Offer practical strategies for

introducing mindfulness into regular

tasks. From mindful dining to mindful walking, present simple yet effective ways for readers to create a thoughtful lifestyle.

Creating relaxation rituals: Guide readers in building relaxing practices. Whether it's a nightly routine before bed or a momentary stop throughout a hectic day, promote the formation of customized relaxation practices.

Real-Life Resonance: Personal Stories of Mind-Body Transformation

Share real-life accounts of individuals who experienced a positive shift in their fertility journey by recognizing the mind-body link. Humanize the science, making it relevant and inspirational for readers.

3.2 ALTERNATIVE THERAPIES

Beyond Conventional Paths:

Exploring Alternative Avenues

Acupuncture:

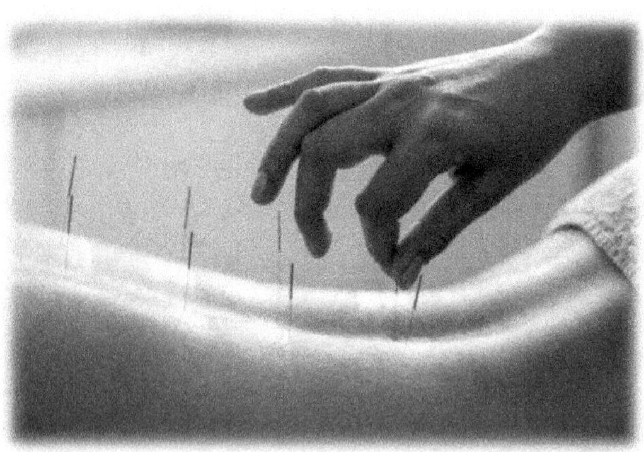

The Art of Energetic Balance

Demystify acupuncture by examining its ancient roots and current uses in improving fertility. Provide a scientific context for acupuncture's impact on egg quality, reinforced with stories or testimonies.

Herbal Supplements:

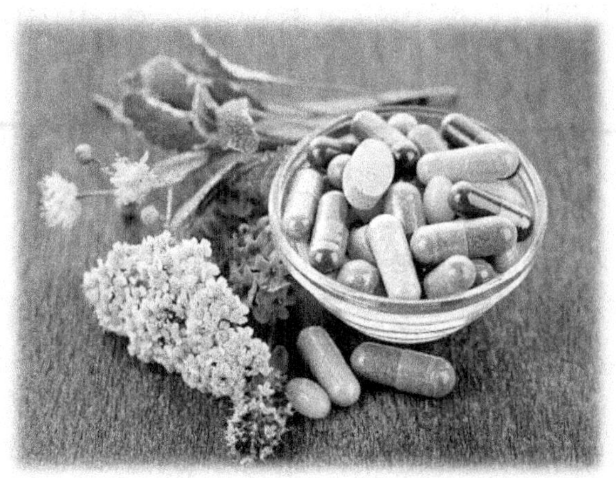

Nature's Nourishment for Fertility

Navigate the terrain of herbal

supplements renowned for their good

effects on fertility. From Vitex to

Maca root, describe their possible

advantages while retaining a reader-friendly tone. Include success stories or testimonials to boost reader confidence.

A Holistic Symphony: Blending Alternative Therapies Showcase the synergistic potential of mixing various alternative medicines. Offer ideas about how readers might develop a tailored holistic approach by mixing acupuncture, herbal supplements, and mindfulness

activities.

Reader's Exploration: A Personalized Holistic Journey

Navigating alternative therapies responsibly: Provide advice on

approaching alternative treatments

ethically. Encourage readers to check

with healthcare experts and

specialists before adopting these

methods in their reproductive

journey.

Curating a personalized holistic

plan: Empower readers to design

their own customized, comprehensive

strategies. Offer templates or

recommendations for combining

alternative therapies, enabling

freedom for individual preferences.

Voices of Transformation:

Testimonials on Alternative

Therapies: Share testimonials or success stories from individuals who have embraced alternative therapy in their fertility quest. Highlight the diversity of pathways, highlighting that each trip is unique. By integrating scientific insights with accessible anecdotes, this section strives to explain the comprehensive pathways available for boosting egg quality.

It urges readers to explore the transforming possibilities of the mind-body connection and alternative therapies on their reproductive journey.

CHAPTER 4

ADVANCED FERTILITY TECHNOLOGIES AND TREATMENTS

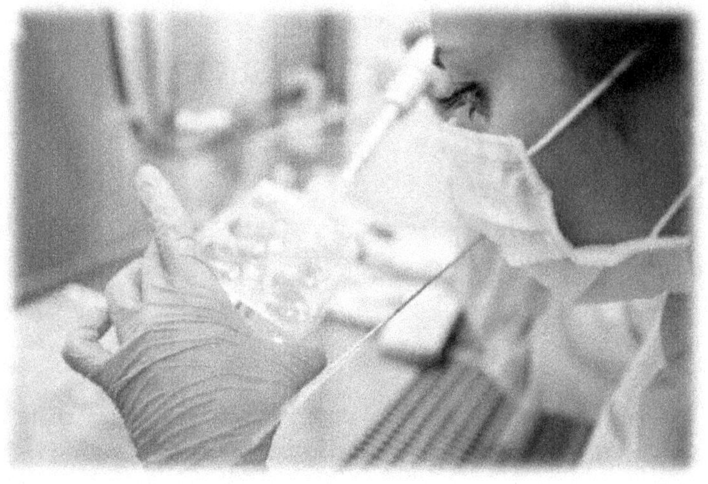

In the ever-evolving world of fertility, developments in technology offer doors to possibilities formerly

believed unachievable. This chapter goes into the domain of advanced fertility technologies and treatments, offering light on the complicated procedures of assisted reproductive technologies (ART) and the proactive decision of egg freezing for future fertility.

4.1 ASSISTED REPRODUCTIVE TECHNOLOGIES (ART)

Decoding the Tapestry of ART:

From Hope to Conception

In Vitro Fertilization (IVF):

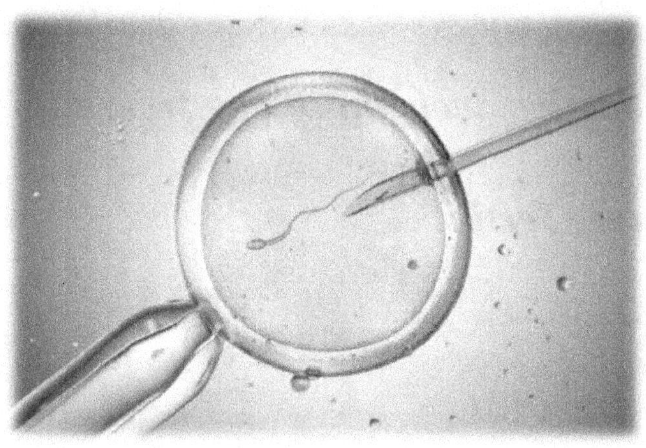

A Pioneering Journey Start with demystifying the intricate world of IVF. Break down the operation into manageable parts, using accessible language and even visual assistance. Illustrate the function of IVF in addressing issues linked to poor egg quality.

Navigating the IVF Landscape: A Q&A Exploration Address typical issues and inquiries pertaining to IVF.

Craft a Q&A section that anticipates the apprehensions readers could have. Provide clear, straightforward responses to demystify the process further.

Beyond IVF: Exploring Additional ART Procedures Expand the debate to incorporate additional ART treatments. From intracytoplasmic sperm injection (ICSI) to gamete intrafallopian transfer (GIFT), give insights into the multiplicity of ART techniques accessible. Share real-life tales of individuals who achieved success with these methods.

Reader's Perspective: Understanding and Embracing ART

Personalizing the IVF Experience: Guide readers in customizing their IVF journey. Discuss factors such as finding the best clinic, understanding success rates, and accepting the

emotional element of the procedure.

ART Success Stories: A Beacon of

Hope Share inspirational success

stories from individuals who achieved

conception via ART. Illuminate the

different roads to success, conveying

the concept that reproductive

journeys are as unique as the

individuals starting on them.

6.2 EGG FREEZING AND PRESERVATION

Preserving Potential: A Proactive Step in Fertility

Egg Freezing:

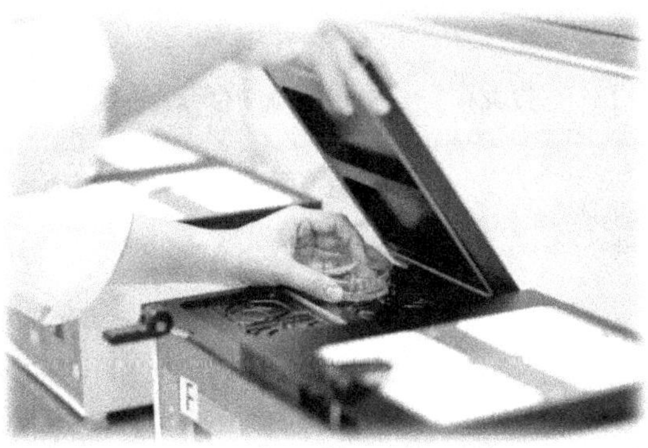

A Contemporary Perspective Unpack the notion of egg freezing, presenting the science underlying the procedure. Explore the reasons someone may make this choice, whether due to job aspirations, medical considerations, or personal preferences.

Benefits and Considerations:

Navigating the decision Delve into the benefits and possible issues related to egg freezing. Offer a balanced viewpoint, emphasizing both the empowering elements of retaining fertility options and the considerations that come with them.

Voices of Choice: Personal Stories of Egg Freezing Share anecdotes of folks who have opted for egg freezing. Include stories that include varied motives, from career-focused choices to proactive family planning. Illustrate the multiplicity of pathways and decisions within the field of fertility preservation.

READER'S CONSIDERATION: NAVIGATING CHOICES FOR FUTURE FERTILITY

Decision-Making Guide: Is Egg Freezing Right for You? Provide a decision-making guide to help readers determine if egg freezing corresponds with their objectives and circumstances. Offer introspective

questions and thoughts to help in the

decision-making process.

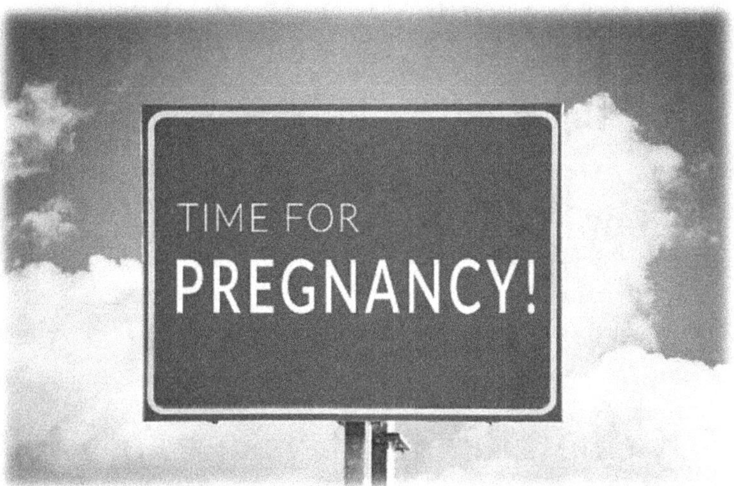

Fertility Planning Beyond the Present: Encourage readers to envision their own journey beyond the present time. Discuss how egg freezing fits within a larger spectrum of family planning, highlighting the proactive character of this decision. By demystifying the nuances of ART and presenting egg freezing as a proactive decision, this chapter strives to empower readers with knowledge and alternatives. It encourages

individuals to explore sophisticated

reproductive technologies with a

feeling of awareness and agency,

boosting optimism and informed

decision-making.

CHAPTER 5

SUCCESS STORIES AND REAL-LIFE EXPERIENCE

Embarking on a reproductive journey is a very personal experience, generally distinguished by tenacity, optimism, and, finally, success. In this chapter, we dig into the real-world tales that breathe life into the reproductive landscape personal testimonials that mirror the victories of individuals who overcome hurdles and professional perspectives that give a multidimensional understanding of fertility advancements.

5.1 PERSONAL TESTIMONIALS

Inspirational Narratives: Triumphs in the Face of Challenges

Diverse Fertility Journeys:

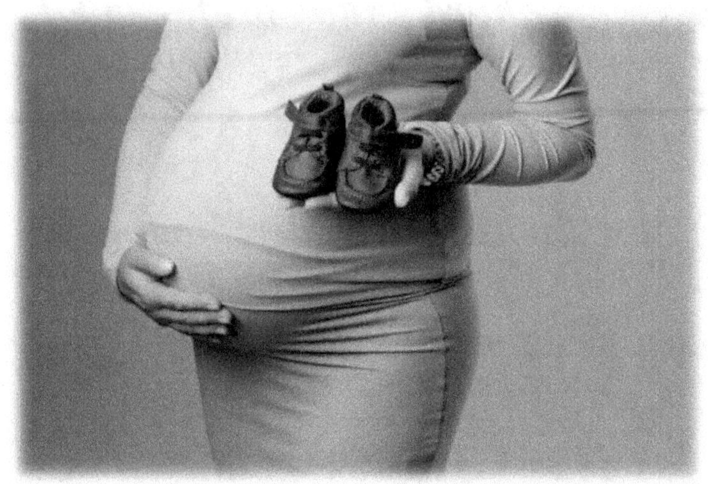

A Tapestry of Hope Introduce a

collection of personal testimonies,

guaranteeing variety in backgrounds,

experiences, and outcomes. Highlight

stories of success over hardship,

focusing on varied problems such as age-related reproductive concerns, medical complexity, and unexplained infertility.

Couples' Perspectives: A Shared Journey Share anecdotes from couples who tackled the fertility journey together. Explore the dynamics of mutual support, emotional resilience, and the transforming potential of tackling

obstacles as a unified front.

Single Parent Success Stories:

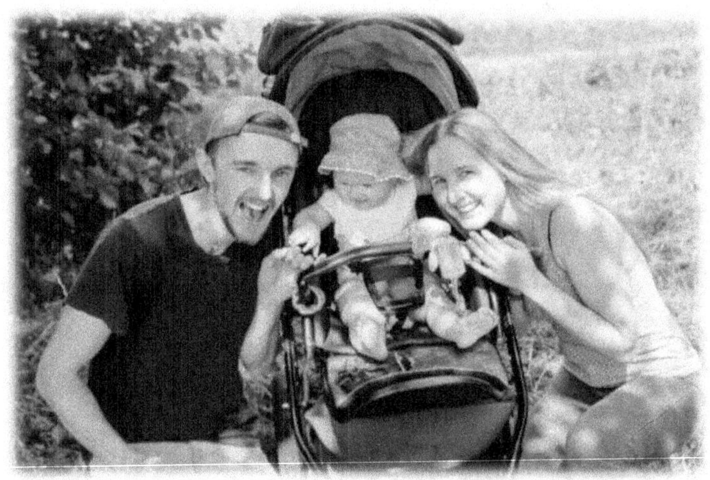

The Power of Choice Feature tales of

individuals who choose the route of

single parenthood Illuminate the different reasons behind this choice and applaud the bravery and tenacity of people who built their own unique roads to motherhood. Reader's

Reflection: Finding Hope in Shared Experiences

Empathy and Connection: Relating to Others' Journeys Guide readers in connecting with the common experiences of persons in the testimonies. Encourage empathy and compassion, establishing a sense of community among individuals managing their own reproductive issues.

Reflective Journaling: A Personalized Approach Provide opportunities for reflective journaling, enabling readers to explore their own feelings and thoughts as they connect with the different stories. Emphasize the

therapeutic value of introspection and

self-discovery.

5.2 EXPERT INSIGHTS

Holistic Perspectives: Insights from

Fertility Specialists

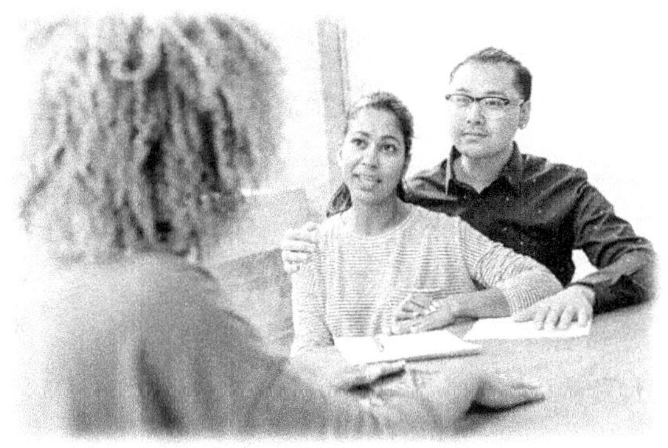

Medical Perspectives: Breakthroughs in Assisted Reproductive Technologies (ART) Feature insights from reproductive professionals about new developments in ART. Discuss developments in technology, creative therapies, and success stories that reflect the dynamic landscape of assisted reproduction.

Psychological Aspects: Navigating the emotional terrain Explore the psychological elements of fertility breakthroughs. Include comments from psychologists and counselors on coping methods, resilience, and emotional well-being during the fertility process.

Holistic Approaches: Beyond Medicine Present holistic opinions from professionals that mix alternative therapies into reproductive treatments. Discuss the importance of diet, acupuncture, and mind-body practices in boosting fertility and general well-being.

Reader's Inquiry: Navigating Questions and Seeking Answers

Interactive Q&A: Addressing Common Concerns Create an interactive Q&A section, answering frequent questions readers might have after engaging with the personal testimonies and professional views.

Provide straightforward and simple replies, giving advice and reassurance.

Seeking Professional Guidance:

Encouraging Consultation Emphasize the necessity of receiving expert counsel adapted to specific situations. Provide tools and recommendations on choosing reliable fertility doctors and support services.

By mixing personal testimony and expert perspectives, this chapter tries to explain the different dimensions of the reproductive journey. It enables readers to discover peace, inspiration, and vital information as they travel their own pathways toward achieving their dreams of motherhood.

<u>CONCLUSION</u>

As we reach the end of this reproductive breakthrough guide, it's time to reflect on the important ideas, successes, and insights that have unfolded in the prior chapters. This conclusion seeks to summarize the essential insights, enhance your understanding of fertility, and set the foundation for a positive and educated path ahead.

SUMMARIZE KEY TAKEAWAYS

Focus on Egg Quality: A Cornerstone of Fertility Success

The Central Role of Egg Quality

Recap the critical importance of egg quality in the fertility equation. Summarize the science underpinning egg formation, highlighting the important phases and genetic aspects that impact quality. Lifestyle Impact

on Fertility Reinforce the influence of

lifestyle decisions on fertility

Summarize the role of diet, stress

management, and holistic methods in

enhancing overall reproductive

health.

Navigating Fertility Technologies

Summarize the important issues about assisted reproductive technology, egg freezing, and alternative medicines. Provide a clear summary of the choices accessible to those seeking fertility help.

Quick-Reference Guide: Your Fertility Companion

A Quick Reference to Essential Tips:

Offer a short guide that readers may resort to for quick insights and reminders. Include realistic recommendations for lifestyle modifications, food choices, and considerations while researching reproductive treatments.

Looking Ahead Embrace Optimism:

Your fertility journey continues.

A Positive Perspective on the Journey: Encourage readers to approach their fertility journey with positivity and resilience. Emphasize that every individual's journey is unique and loaded with possibilities for growth and success.

Recommended Resources for

Further Exploration: Provide a selected list of supplementary resources, such as books, websites, and support groups, where readers may obtain further knowledge and connect with others on similar journeys.

Acknowledgment of Support: You're not alone. Reiterate that help is accessible, whether from experts, support groups, or loved ones.

Acknowledge the fortitude it takes to

go on a fertility journey and offer

sympathy for the hardships involved.

Closing Note: Your Wishes for the Future:

Warm Wishes for the Path Ahead:
Conclude with genuine best wishes

for readers as they continue their

reproductive quest. Express trust in

their capacity to overcome problems

and enjoy accomplishments, whatever shape they may take. Author's

Commitment: A Continued Resource

Affirm your commitment to providing an ongoing resource for people seeking information, assistance, and support in their fertility journey.